I See You

Observations from the ICU

A Caregiver's Journey

Monica Bhide

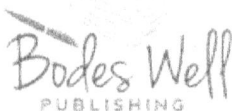

Bodes Well
PUBLISHING

This book is dedicated to our courageous and loving sons, Jai and Arjun. It was your love and the light in your eyes that kept us going. We are both blessed to be your parents.

Contents

How It All Begins, and Where Will It All End? 1

The Only Rule of the ICU 6

Advice 9

Enduring Powerlessness 11

Envision a Rose 13

Pity..16

Panic 18

Seriously: No More Perspective 21

Time 23

Directives 25

Man Versus Machine...27

Family 30

The Ones Who Come and the Ones Who Don't 36

The Myth 38

Happiness Is 41

Terror..43

Permission 46

Vulnerability...48

Acceptance 50

Do Prayers Matter? 53

Pushing the Hurt...55

Who Saves Whom?..58

Out of the Mouths of Babes 61

Does Positive Visualization Work? 64

The Harmony of Rhythm 66

Gifts of Coffee Versus Tea...................................... 68

Who Is in the Bed? 70

All That Glitters 72

The Tunnel 74

Did You Hear the Song?... 80

The Lady with the Ice Cream 82

Well-Meaning Advice.. 85

The Doctors and Their Science 90

Can It Be Taught? 93

Lifelines... 96

A Funny Moment 99

The Global ICU.. 100

Feeding the Ones You Love................................... 102

Darkness 108

Night Terrors 110

All Humans... 112

Hope.. 114

Energy.. 116

Bitten 117

Bathroom Break 119

Protest.. 122

Depends on the Destination.................................. 125

Normal 127

Wild Horses 129

If These Walls Could Talk 131

A Little Knowledge... 134

ICU Amnesia...136

Monitoring the Monitors 139

Fashion in the ICU...141

The Body Does What the Body Does! 143

Bite-Sized Blessings..145

It Is Always the Food 147

Why Me?...149

What Matters 151

The "No Crying" Rule 153

In the Darkness 156

The Moment...158

Movement...162

Why Walk?..163

The World We Live In 165

When Rules Don't Matter 167

The Meaning Is Yours 169

One Sock at a Time...171

Who Is Ill?..173

How Do You Do It?..175

Ice Packs...177

How to Heal..179

Hiding in Plain Sight..182

Finding Peace 184

This and Only This 186

The Three Ladies of Fate 188

True Sight 191

The Hands 193

Of Curses and Blessings......................................195

What Do You See? 198

Best Blessing Ever..201
Check Out 204

Resources 207
Acknowledgements...209
About the Author..211
Also by Monica Bhide 213

The birth of this book

This book was born out of the perfect storm: my healthy husband's sudden deathly illness and my desperate, almost obsessive need to find something good in the situation. My soul friends, Jennifer and Domenica, organized a GoFundMe campaign that not only made this book possible, but also made it possible for me to keep working while I tended to my seriously ailing husband. To honor all those who have helped make this work possible, we are donating multiple copies (one for every person who funded the campaign) of this book to the local hospital that saved my husband's life.

A note from my husband, Sameer Bhide

*"I never wanted to have a major illness! Who does? That said, I am grateful that Monica has taken this devastating experience for me and our family and turned it into a book designed to help others in need. Monica and I truly hope that this book will be helpful to anyone who finds themselves in a difficult medical crisis. "*Sameer Bhide

How It All Begins, and
Where Will It All End?

Our family recently faced a life-changing medical emergency: my husband experienced a massive brain bleed and clot. As the doctors, nurses, and other hospital staff worked endlessly to save his life, I was, as a caregiver, on the sidelines. Feelings of helplessness, grief, sadness, and frustration found a home in my heart. During the time of his hospitalization and now, during post-op care, I find myself reaching again and again for the only thing that gives me great comfort: books. For some people, comfort is found in music, or meditation, or walking, or yoga, or rock climbing, or self-medication(!). For me, it always has been and always will be books. I found myself reading everything from favorites such as *When Breath Becomes Air* to more contemporary releases like *Into the Water* by Paula Hawkins. I read books about my husband's life-threatening illness, about finding motivation during hard times, about how to care for yourself while caring for others. During endless hours in waiting rooms, I read what felt like every magazine available.

I wrote a blog post years ago, wondering if my current profession—food writing—even matters. The responses to it surprised me then. But nothing surprised me more than what happened when massive tragedy hit home. I wasn't able to cook or feed my family as I wanted, yet I found myself, late at night, reaching for the cookbooks on my nightstand. Just going through them comforted me, provided solace, and made me think of happier times. I began to bookmark recipes I would cook when things settled down. They gave me hope . . . that things *would* settle down.

Yet as much as I read when my own world collapsed, I stopped writing. My friends, my mentor, and my father constantly told me to keep a journal, but at first I scorned the idea. How could they tell me to keep writing when everything seemed to be going up in flames? And then, slowly, I realized what was giving me comfort was *words*. Words others had written during times of great turmoil. And some not written during times of turmoil. But all those words offered me great relief during a heartbreaking time. Getting lost in a good mystery to avoid dealing with medical what-ifs for an hour was a blessing. Even if just for an hour.

My first entry in my journal was this one:

> *It is hard to describe how I feel in the ICU. I go from panic to anxiety to peace to sadness all within the span of an hour. I am tired of people telling me to be strong, or that I am strong. Strong is a difficult place to be. I stand strong when I am in denial. Mostly. Sometimes I stand strong in faith, but that is rare. Mostly I stand strong in*

terror. It is quite a lesson to learn that we cannot control anything. The Universe does, indeed, decide what happens when and to whom.

I pondered this question for months, day in and day out. In the ICU, shivering in the parking lot at two in the morning, sitting at my husband's bedside at four a.m., filling out financial aid forms for my son's college applications: What is the point of it all if we can be certain of nothing?

I guess the answer is so simple that it is annoying. The ICU made me understand that there is ONLY NOW, there is only the present moment. There is no point obsessing over the past and no point being anxious over an uncertain future.

It also reminds me to be grateful for what I have today, as fleeting as today may be. It is what is here that matters. What is gone or what is coming isn't important, certain, or even valuable.

Writing down my own pain gave it a home outside my heart; it gave me support from within, made me feel less overwhelmed.

Today, I humbly offer you my observations, as a caregiver, in the high energy-filled, anxiety-provoking world of the ICU.

I wish that no one would ever need this book. But if you find that you do, I hope it helps you.

I want this book to hold your hand. I want this to be your words, your experience, and your inner guide to help you as much or as little as you need.

I just want to tell you one thing before you read on: There is always light. Always. No matter how dark it seems, there is light. Just remember that. Always.

At the end of every note, I have added a small section for you to write your own reflections should you choose to do so. If not, do not worry. I do believe that writing things down helps us heal, as it takes the pain out of us. However, it is your choice to use this book as it suits your needs.

(Please note: I have purposely left out some detailed information about my husband's illness to protect his privacy.)

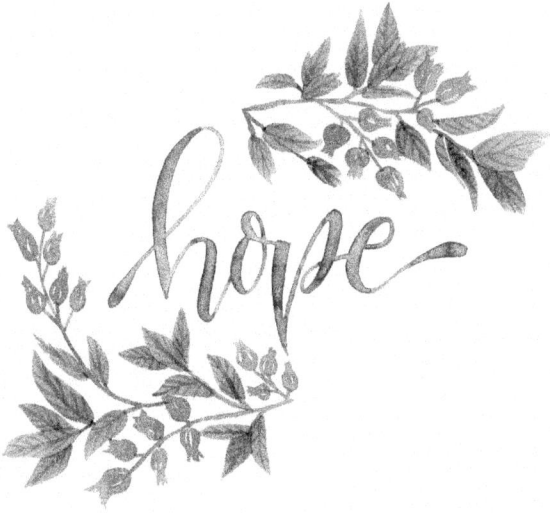

The Only Rule of the ICU

Little did I realize that these words would carry me through every hour of our close to thirty days in the ICU:

"Bad things happen quickly. Good things take time."

Dr. X., a brilliant physician who oversees my husband Sameer's care, tells me this the first time he sees me in the ICU. He comes into the room like a wild breeze. He speaks to the staff using words that I can barely spell—medications, dosages, updates of his condition on the hour. I can tell the staff not only love him, they hold him in very high regard.

"He never forgets anything," one of the senior nurses tells me. "Never. He has so many patients he sees, yet he always remembers everything."

I watch him as he comes and goes from our room—each time reminding me to have patience with everything. "It takes time."

I wonder if we have time. I panic at the intense buzzing noises, blinking signs, constant announcements, incessant emergencies, the nurses reacting almost every second in the ICU. The sights and sounds make me feel like the clock is ticking. The ICU is cold, frigid, surreal. The situation seems impossible as I watch the staff try to save his life. It could all end at any moment.

Then there are moments when I just focus on his face: I see him breathing. I see his chest moving up and down with each lifesaving breath. I hold his hand. It is warm. Perhaps we do have time.

My nerves take a beating with each ticking second. I learn to try and breathe through the day. To catch myself when I feel the panic setting in. To see him breathe and then say out loud to myself: *We have time.*

Your thoughts

_____

_____

_____

_____

_____

_____

_____

_____

_____

_____

_____

Advice

An important piece of advice I received in the ICU came from a dear friend whom I have known for a long, long time. She suffered a devastating illness. I am writing this here with her permission.

"Any crisis like this results in change—to the person who experiences it directly, and to loved ones and caregivers who experience it directly too, but in a different way. There's an old expression that applies here: 'Pay now or pay later,' but essentially, while time and physical healing will help to some degree in the overall emotional 'recovery,' in my experience, those things aren't enough. I do hope that if he and you aren't already getting some counseling, that you will consider it— even if it begins with support groups."

I was sure none of us needed counseling. I was so sure. Even after I read her message, I thought, *Why would we need counseling? I know he is going to survive (no matter what the doctors say) and all will be well.*

Little did I realize that the very nature of a trauma like this is, well, traumatic. I found myself suffering relentless nightmares, moments of dread in the middle of the day, and just the inability to sit still for fear of having to actually think about the situation.

Then, one afternoon, a group of women came to visit me. They were previous patients of this neuro ICU and had survived. They began to tell me their experiences, how hard it was on them and their loved ones. One shared her experience of going to a rehab center after her illness. It suddenly occurred to me that I needed to not just focus on now, but to think of my husband's wellness in the future and the kind of rehab he would need. Their realistic yet uplifting chat made me direct my energy forward instead of being panic-stricken each moment.

I do admit that after that encounter, I took my friend's advice literally and talked to most everyone in the ICU waiting room. Most of the chatter was banal, but there was an underlying camaraderie. We were all in this together. We reminded each other that "we got this." "Ain't no illness bad enough," said an older woman waiting in the ICU with me.

Yes, we got this.

Your thoughts

Enduring Powerlessness

A friend who is recovering from cancer heard what happened and sent me a note telling me he understood what it was like to endure powerlessness.

It took me a while to understand that phrase: *Endure powerlessness.*

How does one do that?

How do you endure something so devastating?

As I sit and watch the nurses change tubes, add more medication, change the room temperature, I see that they have some power to change things. We have that. Perhaps that is not power but hope.

It would be a lot harder to endure hopelessness than powerlessness, I decide.

For the moment, that is my truth.

Ask me again in three hours or so.

Your thoughts

_____

_____

_____

_____

_____

_____

_____

_____

_____

_____

_____

_____

Envision a Rose

The ICU doesn't permit flowers, yet a lot of kind friends buy flowers and place them in the waiting room outside.

I remember one particular bouquet of white roses. There were droplets of water on the petals. I hadn't been out in a while and had no idea if it had been raining or if it was simply dew on the roses. I remember seeing the flowers and, lost in my own pain, I wondered if flowers cry, or do they just bear the burden of the rain?

I asked my father, who is not only an insightful man but a beautiful poet. He began by asking me what I had seen when I'd traveled to a part of Delhi that houses the graves of many Sufi saints. I tried to remember. (I have to say that it was hard, as I was swaying between severe anxiety and attempting to stay calm.) I remembered: I saw a lot of people praying over the graves, but mostly I recalled people crying over them.

Dad said, then, just as the graves of the saints bear the despair and grief of the world, the flowers bear the burden of the dew. It is not only their privilege—they have the strength to do it.

We have the strength to bear our burdens. If the gentle flower can bear the burden of the dew, our powerful souls can bear the burden of the grief that we are facing here today.

Your thoughts

_____

_____

_____

_____

_____

_____

_____

_____

_____

_____

_____

Pity

Under the chilling breeze of the vent, I sit and blow gently on my fingers to keep them from turning blue. It is a thing I have. It has a long name. But right now it is not important. Right now, I am focused on the new nurse who is being trained to give Sameer some medication.

What I have noticed again and again here in the ICU is how the eyes of the staff sparkle. They don't have pity as they look at him or at me. Their eyes have resilience. It gives me great solace.

Only those who come in from the outside have pity in their eyes for those who are suffering here. They do not see what those of us on the inside do: The people who work here are determined to heal; there is so much strength in their sheer willpower, and such uplifting energy in their presence. Pity implies we are powerless. Pity is a judgment without knowing what the outcome can be.

The ones inside the embrace of the ICU—the patients, their families, the staff—have all learned, I think, that pity has no place here. Only strength does.

Your thoughts

_____

_____

_____

_____

_____

_____

_____

_____

_____

_____

_____

_____

Panic

I have decided, in all my wisdom, that I will only panic if the head nurse panics.

I watch her every day when she comes in to make the rounds. I watch her like a hawk. She checks on him, every day, and then turns to me and says, "Miracles happen here every day. I have seen them with my own eyes."

I think perhaps she is just using these words to soothe me. I wonder if she really believes them. Then, one day, I ask her. "How do you keep from panicking? How do you not break down with all this illness surrounding you?"

She tells me she used to work at a burn unit. "After working there, this seems much less traumatic."

Perspective, as they say, is everything.

"I stay sane by leaving here when my shift is over. I see you here all the time. You need to leave for a few hours and come back. It will help keep the panic at bay," she advises.

I usually take direction well. But this time, I hesitate. I decide to keep watching her expressions instead. If she panics, I will. If not, all will be well.

Your thoughts

_____

_____

_____

_____

_____

_____

_____

_____

_____

_____

_____

Seriously: No More Perspective

My friend is driving me home one night from the hospital. We get into a massive car accident, a first for both of us. Luckily, no one is hurt.

Her car is totaled. We get out, with the help of some kind passersby, and try to steady ourselves. A young man on the scene offers me advice. "I hope you are okay. Accidents always set perspective."

I am tired of damn perspective.

Perhaps, I have what my friend Jennifer calls perspective fatigue. I need a little less perspective right now and a little more peace.

Your thoughts

_____

_____

_____

_____

_____

_____

_____

_____

_____

_____

_____

Time

The night before my husband was admitted to the ICU, he was talking to a travel agent about booking a vacation for the summer. We wanted to take our son to Europe before he left for college. Now I sit here with his phone in my hands and receive the agent's text messages asking if she should book the tickets and what dates work the best.

Time and date, she asks.

I want to respond with a time and date, yet my fingers hesitate. Should I be bold and fearless and optimistic and book tickets while our future hangs by the whirring of the respirator? Or should I cancel plans, not yet final, and see what happens?

I text her and say wait. It isn't time yet.

Your thoughts

_____

_____

_____

_____

_____

_____

_____

_____

_____

_____

_____

Directives

Late one night, one of the nurses is doing her best to keep Sameer alive. She has been toiling tirelessly with medication, checking his breathing tube, monitoring his heart rate. Suddenly, she turns to me and asks, "Does he have an advance medical directive?"

It's two a.m. The room goes from being chilly to downright frozen.

"If he doesn't, it's okay. I am just checking," she says cheerfully and goes back to work.

It is, after all, the ICU. A place where lives are saved.

And lost.

Your thoughts

_____

_____

_____

_____

_____

_____

_____

_____

_____

_____

_____

Man Versus Machine

I open my sleepy eyes and see Dr. X. standing next to Sameer's bed. It is around five a.m. and still pitch-black outside. The large windows behind me are dark. The beeps, the sounds of the ICU, seem familiar, so I try not to panic as I wonder what the kind doctor is doing, standing so still. He never stands still. I can feel the pressure in my chest.

He is studying his patient, intently. He isn't doing anything—it would seem. But as my eyes open wide and the remnants of the night's sleep disappear, I watch the doctor quietly.

He is doing something, it finally occurs to me, that I haven't seen many others do. Instead of just focusing on all the machines and their readings and beeps, he is also observing Sameer. He bends down for a closer look at his eyes. He then listens to Sameer's heart.

I watch him as he steps back and places one hand on his chin and rubs it. He looks at the monitors again. Then checks Sameer again.

Yes, he is exactly as you would picture a brilliant doctor to be.

Finally, he pages the night nurse. He doesn't need to. She is ready and waiting behind him. It occurs to me that she knows him so well. She anticipates his moves.

He turns to her and smiles. It is five in the morning and she is ready with her computer turned on and she begins typing as he in his kindest, gentlest voice orders a whole bunch of new tests.

Finally, he turns to me and says, "I think I know what is wrong. We will try to fix it."

My mouth opens to say thanks, but he is gone in the blink of an eye.

Can this instinct be taught? I wonder.

Your thoughts

_____

_____

_____

_____

_____

_____

_____

_____

_____

_____

_____

_____

Family

I am sitting in the ICU waiting room as Sameer is having a procedure.

Our closest friends haven't left our side for weeks. They don't ask permission to come. They show up. They sit and hold my hand. His hand. They feed my kids.

Today: My sister is here, as my friends take a much-needed afternoon off. She and I are talking about what seems totally irrelevant—the weather. How does it even matter what happens outside when the one you love is breathing with the help of machines? But we talk as if it is purposeful. Perhaps, I think, it is my brain's way of avoiding total shutdown. We try to focus on the rain outside, on the changing weather, on the pattern differences between the West Coast (where she lives) and here on the East Coast. The conversation actually helps calm my nerves.

Suddenly the usually quiet waiting room becomes a stage for drama. A large family sitting beside us is having a huge argument about current, unsettling politics and the incessant media coverage of every presidential tweet. "Our mother is dying inside, and all you can do is discuss politics? And fight right now?" says a young man in the group.

He gets up, shoots us an apologetic look, wipes a tear from his eyes, and leaves the room.

The family goes back to talking politics. My sister and I continue to discuss the weather. All irrelevant. But, I wonder later, is this a survival technique? For me it was the weather, for them it was politics. A way to give the brain some relief.

Your thoughts

_____

_____

_____

_____

_____

_____

_____

_____

_____

_____

_____

_____

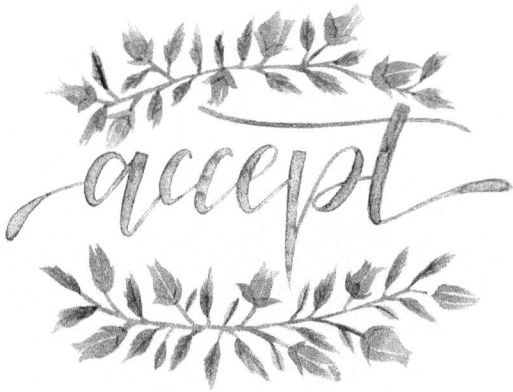

The Ones Who Come
and the Ones Who Don't

Any crisis brings out people's personalities: the good, the bad, the ugly, and the "please leave now before I commit felony murder."

We had a steady stream of visitors, and there were many times I could not talk to anyone. Most stayed and understood. There were a few who didn't. And then, the hardest of the lot were the ones who wanted to offer me advice on what to do and what not to do—regardless of how much they knew or did not know about the situation.

There were some people I just did not want to see. I could not handle their overly inquisitive questions, their probing words and their dire predictions of the future.

I had to ask a friend, in all seriousness, to prepare some canned answers for me so that I did not curse people out. To the people telling me how Sameer's treatment should or should not proceed, my automatic response became: "Thank you so much for that great advice. I will be sure to check in with the doctor/neurosurgeon/etc."

I wish I could just be all politically correct here and tell you that people reacted well to my answers and that I did all the right things. I know I made mistakes in how I handled things during the stress. However, I also know that if I had listened to every wannabe therapist telling me how to cope or what to do for my husband, I would have gone crazy.

Your thoughts

_____

_____

_____

_____

_____

_____

_____

_____

_____

_____

_____

The Myth

Before my husband's major illness, I was a planner: I made lists, I marked things off my to-do list, I worried about things big and small with equal intensity. Then one day, my husband ends up in the ICU, I have a massive car accident, another kid's mom accidentally feeds my child food he is allergic to . . . all in the same six weeks.

It occurs to me as I sit in the ICU that the one thing we humans *think* we have is control.

What freaking control?

Don't get me wrong: I am all for planning life, making to-do lists, but after all this, I have realized that my lists, and dreams, and all that can be is just that. It *can* be. It isn't what *is*.

I realized the only thing I could control in that ICU was my reaction. My attitude. My thoughts—with a lot of help from friends.

"Breathe. No matter what the report says, you try to find your center," one dear friend advises.

"Take short walks, go outside. I will stay with him," my sister says. As hard as it is, I leave for a few minutes to go try and find that reclusive center and mindfulness.

"Go easy on yourself, you are handling a lot," says another dear friend, advising me to do a few minutes of meditation throughout the day.

All I can do is be present, be focused and loving toward all those who are trying to help, to my children who need me and are hurting and to myself.

That is it. I realize that is all any of us can really do in a time of massive crisis: control our mindset.

Who has control? I don't know. And today, sitting in the ICU, I am not sure I care to debate the existence of God or the Universe or whomever.

I just focus on now: one mindful breath at a time.

Your thoughts

_____

_____

_____

_____

_____

_____

_____

_____

_____

_____

_____

Happiness Is

If I cannot find any solace, joy, happiness, peace in what I have now and in this moment, then I have nothing.

I used to think I would be happy when I became a writer, then it became when I was a *paid* writer, then a *known* writer—see where this is going?

After what happened, it hit me that my only chance at happiness is with what I have right now. A loving husband who is still breathing—all I have is this moment to be happy.

It is a hard pill to swallow that the happiness we so crave lies not outside and beyond, but inside and now.

What if this is all there is?

What if?

Your thoughts

Terror

I learn quickly in the ICU that humor is the most-loved healing tool. It has to be, right? *Laughter heals*, the doctors keep telling me.

Our friends come in and tell sweet stories of their time with Sameer: his intense focus on making us love his favorite musical artist, his ability to create funny top ten lists of all our times together, his obsessive love of desserts. We make a list of everything we are doing wrong in the ICU (one of us snored so loudly we frightened the night nurse; we couldn't figure out how to convert a simple chair into a bed there) and we laugh even though we are all shaken to our cores.

My friend V., who is clumsy to say the least, has made a huge effort not to step on all the wires that surround Sameer's bed. We laugh about that. It isn't callous. It isn't mean. We are trying to normalize a situation that is beyond our capacity.

"When he wakes up, we will tell him you did not trip on a single wire!" I say to her. She laughs. Then she goes up to him and says, "I am driving your car. I have your keys here. Come on. Wake up now. I have your car, for God's sake. I can damage it. You know how clumsy I am."

She leaves the room in tears.

I sit on the chair and watch him. When the laughter subsides, terror returns.

He still isn't awake.

Your thoughts

_____

_____

_____

_____

_____

_____

_____

_____

_____

_____

_____

_____

Permission

As the days turned to nights and the nights turned to days, the endless cycle of worry began to chisel away at my spirit.

I took walks, I meditated, I breathed (sometimes even mindfully).

Then, one day, sitting in the cafeteria at five in the morning, I began to cry. It was the first time I had cried since we had entered this ICU weeks ago.

I cried and cried and cried for what had happened, for what could happen, for what may not happen. I let the fear out, I purged it from my system.

I literally gave myself permission to weep, not just for him and his illness, but for my children and yes, for myself. I cried.

Then, I went back up to his room and followed my own rule of no crying inside his room and told him about how good the coffee tasted and how much he would love it.

Your thoughts

Vulnerability

I see now that with my tears, I came upon a different emotion: vulnerability. As I cried and cried, I let go of the stoic image I had created for myself, the firm, strong adult who never broke down no matter how hard it got.

The fear had started to paralyze me. Finding strength in the middle of the tempest was hard. Yet in my moment of greatest despair, in my tears, I realized it was okay to weep. Weeping showed me that I cared, that I worried, and most importantly, that while I was vulnerable, I could still go deep inside and find the strength to move forward, one step, one hour, one day at a time.

Your thoughts

_____

_____

_____

_____

_____

_____

_____

_____

_____

_____

_____

_____

Acceptance

Watching someone you love lie in an ICU bed is painful, to say the least. It makes you feel powerless at some level. At first, I thought that when I felt powerless, I was lost, and that I had given up—or worse, that no one could help me.

Then it happened. Late one night, as I watched, my husband's health failed further. His breathing became labored, and despite the best efforts from the doctors, there was no movement in any of his limbs. While their words were supportive, I could see the despair in their eyes. Though they were doing all they could, he was not improving. He had been in a medically induced coma for three weeks now.

That night, I found my powerlessness becoming my path to finding strength in the Universe, in a power bigger than all of us.

The powerlessness forced me to deliberately focus all my thoughts on the great Source. I prayed from a place of least resistance—this prayer was not a plea of desperation. Rather it was a prayer of peace, of being granted the ability to accept what is. I prayed for the doctors who were treating him, for the nurses who watched over him with such care. I prayed all our paths be guided by what was the best for all concerned. I prayed hard for the Universe to help my husband in whatever it was he needed. The prayer became truly a manifestation of accepting the present and being open to whatever the future held. And the recognition that we are guided by an invisible hand of love.

Your thoughts

_____

_____

_____

_____

_____

_____

_____

_____

_____

_____

_____

_____

Do Prayers Matter?

As we watch our loved ones being cared for by doctors and nurses, we sit on the sidelines and try to help. Some pray, some cry, some write, some knit. It isn't easy. When I sat on that cold, hard ICU chair for what seemed like decades, people would text/email/call/walk in and ask how they could help. I always said the same thing: Please pray. I do understand, as my friend Jennifer says, that prayers are not a vending machine where you pop in a particular prayer, and out comes your desired result.

I did not know what the outcome was going to be. What I do know is that the prayers provided comfort during dark nights, when the machines in the ICU buzzed loudly and the nurses paged the doctors in panic. In those times, the prayers helped me hold on for just one more moment.

Your thoughts

Pushing the Hurt

A few weeks into our time at the ICU, Sameer was still in a medically induced coma and I was facing decisions no human should have to make: staring death in the face and wondering what to do about it.

Around noon that day, just as the sun was at its strongest, a young man walked into our ICU room. He was a volunteer chaplain. He asked if I wanted to talk to him. I am not Christian, and even though I am Hindu by birth, I don't really follow organized religion, so I hesitated. He noticed the hesitation and said simply that perhaps we could just chat as two people who want to know each other. I could not say no to his kind demeanor and his sweet and gentle voice.

He had given up a lucrative career in technology to become a priest. He said what he did now brought him great peace. Suddenly, as a career changer myself, I found myself opening up to him a little and talking about the situation at hand.

At some point, I said that I felt like a heavy weight was sitting on my chest. He stood up and said, "I can tell you how to fix that in an instant!"

I froze. *Here it comes. Here comes the speech to join some religion . . .* I remember thinking.

Instead, he asked me to accompany him out to the main corridor, where we found a large blank wall. "Now. Come here. Stand in front of this wall. Push as hard as you can. Stand straight, legs a little apart. Now use your arms and push against that wall. That will cause that weight—also known as anxiety—to break down and shift. You need your energy to pray and heal yourself, not to be weighed down by fear."

I cannot tell you how many times in those months I pushed walls all around the ICU, at home, anywhere I could. The anxiety needed a place to go. To be earthed.

To this day, I am thankful to him for showing me the way to push out the hurt.

Your thoughts

_____

_____

_____

_____

_____

_____

_____

_____

_____

_____

_____

Who Saves Whom?

It is hard to expect a drowning man to throw a line to someone safely on the shore. And yet, that is exactly what I was doing in the ICU. I was hoping beyond hope that my husband, who was dying and in a coma, would open his eyes, reach out and say, "Honey, everything will be okay."

I would hold his hand and hold back my tears.

Then, a few weeks into the ICU stay, I instinctively began to visualize and then verbalize out loud what he would do when he did wake up. We would go for walks, eat our favorite meals, take the kids on vacation. I tried to be the one giving him hope and positive vibes instead of expecting him to save me.

I don't know if he could hear me or not when he was in the coma, but the doctors said they thought he could, so I kept at it. I had one-way discussions with him on everything from the weather, to my son's college decision, to the quality of the coffee in the hospital cafeteria.

He couldn't tell me everything would be okay. But I certainly could tell him that is what we wanted and were praying for every single minute.

Your thoughts

_____

_____

_____

_____

_____

_____

_____

_____

_____

_____

_____

_____

Out of the Mouths of Babes

One Sunday evening, I was sitting in the waiting room while the doctors worked on my husband. A young woman was visiting the hospital with a little girl who could not have been more than four. The two went into the ICU and were there for a little while, then came back and sat down next to me in the waiting room.

"Mama, is this the place where people come to get sick?" the young girl asked her mother.

"No, no. This is where people come to get well," the mother answered.

"Then why is everyone here sick?"

The mother said something about the child needing food and left the waiting room, visibly embarrassed.

After they walked away, I reflected on what the sweet child had said. In her naiveté, she had stated the obvious that no one wanted to admit. No one has a magic wand, or there would be no illness. But equally real were the dedicated people who have made it their life's mission to heal.

Your thoughts

_____

_____

_____

_____

_____

_____

_____

_____

_____

_____

_____

Does Positive Visualization Work?

As I sat vigil for long nights, I talked with several doctors, healers, and friends who suggested that I visualize all the happy times that were and that will be. I saw us together at my son's upcoming school graduation, I saw us laughing and enjoying a new movie, I saw us sitting and eating a meal together as a family.

I did so diligently. Many times, that visualization helped me find my center. Sometimes, I could not finish a session as the panic would set in. At those times, I would get up and go for a walk or push a wall to release my anxiety.

Did my visualizations work to heal him? I don't know. But what I do know is this—if I had not visualized positively, my mind would have gone to the darkest corners there are and stayed there. I would have broken down and not been of much use to him or my children.

Visualization gave me a choice: to exist on the side of hope or the side of darkness.

Your thoughts

The Harmony of Rhythm

On days when the ICU got under my skin, I discovered, quite by accident, something that used to soothe me as a child.

Believe it or not, I went for a walk near my house and found a swing.

Sitting on that swing, with my eyes closed, the cold wind in my hair and my breathing steady, I was back to being ten. Mom and Dad were there in my mind, telling me all would be well. The rhythm of the swing somehow shifted the energy in my body.

Even after Sameer was released from the ICU, I found myself back at the swing every chance I got. The rhythm of peace was mine for the taking. And it was free.

Your thoughts

Gifts of Coffee Versus Tea

For six months, in and post ICU, we received kind gifts from friends and family. One thing I observed—I am a food writer, after all—was that the beverage we received as a gift was tea. No coffee. Always tea.

Is tea the comfort drink and coffee the work drink?

I don't know.

Random thoughts from a tired ICU caregiver.

Your thoughts

_____

_____

_____

_____

_____

_____

_____

_____

_____

_____

_____

_____

Who Is in the Bed?

There came a time when it was getting harder to recognize my husband. He had so many tubes, so many machines attached to him. It was becoming more and more difficult to see the person on the bed. I wondered how this illness would affect him long-term, I worried about his quality of life, I recalled scenes from movies where people wake up from a coma and cannot recognize the people around them.

A friend stopped in one day and when I told her this, she said, "The mirror doesn't stop being a mirror because it has a bit of dust on it. Don't worry. The dust will be removed soon."

Your thoughts

All That Glitters

I wear a pendant of Lord Krishna around my neck. It was a gift from my father, who gave it to me when I turned twenty-one. While I don't follow any organized religion, I love what I know of Lord Krishna—the epitome of love and kindness.

One day, a priest of some repute came for a visit and asked me what I was wearing around my neck. I said, "It is a pendant of Lord Krishna."

"I know who it is. I am just asking you if you are wearing jewelry or if you are wearing faith," he said as he smiled.

I was a bit flustered. His question unnerved me.

Noting the tears in my eyes, he added, "We humans want to see proof of the Universal energy, and then we say we will have faith. It is the other way around. What you are wearing will give you the energy to create and manifest miracles around you. The key is to believe it first." Tears rolled down my cheeks and he added, gently, "It takes a lifetime to have unwavering faith. All I am saying is that the Divine is with you, so try to have faith. Don't get frustrated."

Your thoughts

_____

_____

_____

_____

_____

_____

_____

_____

_____

_____

_____

The Tunnel

I have always believed in the age-old cliché that there is light at the end of tunnel. In fact, I was telling my sister about this saying one night in the ICU. Just before I fell asleep, the nurses were with Sameer, giving him medication, watching his heart rate. "He is getting stronger and soon, he may not need the respirator," one of them said.

Later that night, I woke up sweating from a nightmare that I was in a tunnel and the light was coming at me. It was the headlight of a train. I woke up, startled. My fears were getting the better of me. Even the slightest hope was scaring me. What if the hope was an illusion? What if the light was an illusion?

Shivering, I tried to gather myself. I was frightened.

I paused and thought about the saying again. Instead of thinking that the light is an illusion, what if I flipped my fear on its head: What if it is the tunnel that is the illusion? The light, the hope, is the real thing. The tunnel, the darkness, is temporary.

I reminded myself that he may be off the respirator soon. The light, the reality. The ever-present hope.

I fell back to sleep.

Your thoughts

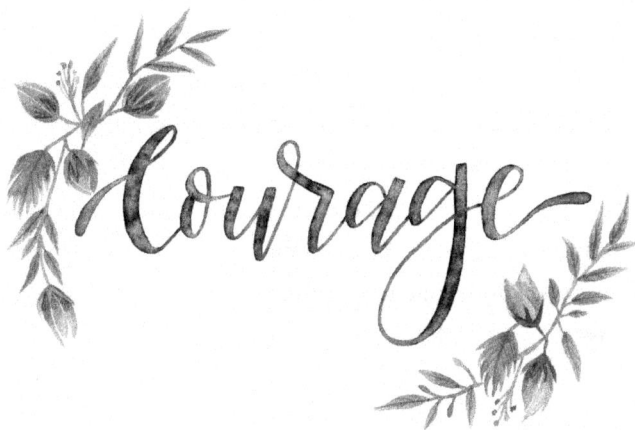

Did You Hear the Song?

There was a woman in the ICU waiting room who always seemed to be humming a prayer or a chant of some sort. I swear I knew she was humming, but it seemed like each time I pointed it out to someone with me, they would insist they couldn't hear anything. She had been there for almost a week, mostly early in the morning, alone. She would come with her family, or people I am assuming were her family, in the evening.

Who was right?

I admit, the chances that I—sleep-deprived, devastated, and afraid— was just hearing things were high. But at first I was annoyed. How could they not hear this hum? What was wrong with them?

Then after a week of arguing, I let it go. Perhaps that hum was just for me. Perhaps she wasn't humming at all, but because I wanted to be near someone who was praying in peace, I was sitting by her side and hearing a quiet prayer.

Sometimes we intellectualize everything. Sometimes it is the heart that hears and not the ears.

I don't know if she actually ever said or hummed anything. But I felt peace sitting by her side; I felt humming. I felt a deep sense of calm knowing that I was going to be okay with the uncertainty. I read once that faith is the evidence of things unseen. In this case, perhaps so—heard or unheard, as the case may be.

Your thoughts

_____

_____

_____

_____

_____

_____

_____

_____

_____

_____

_____

_____

The Lady with the Ice Cream

It is funny how we connect and place stories around those whom we see daily but who are complete strangers.

There was one such woman at the hospital whom I will never ever forget.

Blonde, curly hair, medium height, big blue eyes. She works there. I don't know in what unit or in what capacity, but judging by the color of her scrubs, I would say she's a nurse.

I would pass her many days at five in the morning on the walking bridge that connects the parking lot to the hospital. Occasionally I would see her walking around the cafeteria at lunch. Always smiling, always beaming. She always looked at me with such compassionate eyes. I was grateful for her smile.

One morning, before sunrise, I was walking into the hospital on the walking bridge. It was dark and dreary outside. My heart felt heavy.

I saw her coming out of the hospital building. I will never forget.

She was eating an ice cream cone. A big one. Tears were flowing down her cheeks.

She saw me, smiled weakly, and kept walking. I wanted to run after her, to say *Thank you for always smiling*, to ask what was wrong, to ask her what happened. Instead, I just stood there and watched her walk away with her ice cream.

She was a complete stranger, and yet such a familiar face in my new "regular" world.

At lunch, I asked a friend who was coming to visit to bring ice cream.

Your thoughts

_____

_____

_____

_____

_____

_____

_____

_____

_____

_____

_____

_____

_____

Well-Meaning Advice

Okay, so at some point you will get mad and want to shake this book. Being in the ICU is hard. No matter how calm you are, how strong you are, what a strong believer you are. The environment tests us. It is not an easy place to be.

I had a well-meaning friend who visited frequently and texted me at least twice a day with the words, "Only good can come from this."

My first thought—and admittedly other thoughts, especially when my husband was suffering so badly—was that not only was she delusional, she was being mean. And then I thought she was being so Pollyanna-ish. I was looking for a place to vent my frustration at the situation, and her texts were it. Each time she would send me that text, I would dig my heels in and cuss and say things to myself. Not nice things, mind you. I was cussing. I was angry. I wondered how a dear friend could be so callous in her advice.

This story could have ended any way, and I don't know how it will end for so many. But in this case, I realized the truth of her message after about the thousandth time (or so it felt like) she sent it.

"Only good can come from this" wasn't about the current situation. It was about having faith that a higher power, a higher source of love and compassion, a higher energy, was watching out for us. It has taken me a lifetime to understand that. "Only good can come from this" comes from a simple seed: faith.

It isn't religious faith I am speaking of. It is faith in a Universe that is kind and giving and nurturing. It is believing with every cell in our body that no matter what the circumstances, no matter what happens, when we are ready, we will truly understand and accept: Only good can come from this.

(For the record, I added: *Only good can come from this, twenty years from now.*)

Your thoughts

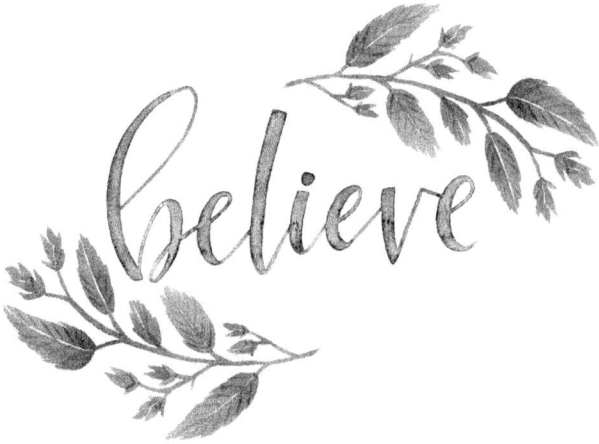

The Doctors and Their Science

No one can quite tell us what caused my husband's illness. I think that single fact was the most disturbing. The doctors could tell us what happened, how they were trying to fix it, what could possibly happen in the future, and, to some extent, what his prognosis was. But no one could tell us what caused it. No one could tell us in certain terms why it happened.

They all had theories. The doctors were amazingly competent, with degrees from big schools. They saved his life. Isn't that all that should have mattered?

But after he left the ICU, I began to research his illness and still could not find a why. The study of brain illnesses is relatively new. Some day they will know why what happened to him happened.

It made me realize that the Universe was forcing my hand: We have to make peace with uncertainty. We may never know.

That is a huge lesson from the ICU. Sometimes we don't know what happens. The best and the brightest minds don't know why and what. All they know is that their job is to heal and to make tomorrow possible. I saw in the staff this ability to live in uncertainty, this ability to adapt in minutes to a rapidly changing situation, this inexplicable hope they all carry that they can make a difference. And that is the energy needed to live and survive in the ICU.

Your thoughts

_____

_____

_____

_____

_____

_____

_____

_____

_____

_____

_____

_____

Can It Be Taught?

My husband's lead acute care doctor was described to me by his nurses as *high energy*. He runs up and down the stairs all day long and nurses half his age cannot keep up with him. He knows every patient's chart from back to front; he knows the exact doses of the many medications he prescribes. It is like he has a photographic memory.

He is teaching medical students as they come in with him on rounds every morning. I see what Dr. X. does as so much more than just doctor. He has sharp instincts: I see him making medication changes based on reading the patient and not just the numbers on the various digital monitors. He soothes my nerves, talks to the nurses when giving them orders for the day. He asks about my children, he wishes my husband good health. He leaves and then comes back to remind me to make sure that I am eating well so I can continue to stay healthy. The students stand mostly in awe. They nod vigorously as he discusses the cases, they blurt out what they think is a diagnosis, and I can see the anxiety on their faces. He listens patiently and then guides them to the conclusions he wants them to reach by pointing out all the details they haven't yet learned to notice and master.

Can this level of medicine be taught, I wonder? Emulated? Perhaps. Replicated? I don't know. I can only pray that the medical students who are walking with him realize his genius lies in equal parts with his experience, his compassion, and his true belief in the sacredness of human life.

Your thoughts

_____

_____

_____

_____

_____

_____

_____

_____

_____

_____

_____

Lifelines

At two in the morning, when the machines in the room would all beep for one reason or another, I found solace in the calm faces of the ICU nurses. I knew they had seen it all, and I figured I would panic only if I saw them panicking.

If they came in and fiddled with the machines and did not look upset, then, I decided, I would not be upset.

Sounds simplistic. It isn't. There is so much stress inside me. As a layperson, I did not understand all the machines. I knew which ones beeped when they ran out of medication or food. This was all great in the daytime when my brain was functioning and able to comprehend what was happening.

The hard part was at night. I would fall asleep in the chair next to his bed and wake up to machines beeping like crazy. I would feel my heart thumping and I would begin counting backwards from twenty-five. The nurses usually showed up before I reached ten. Then, instead of panicking, I would observe their faces. Calm, cool, and doing what needed to be done.

I knew the difference. I had seen them page a doctor at three a.m.

Luckily, most nights, it was just him and me and the relentless nurses of the neuro ICU.

Your thoughts

_____

_____

_____

_____

_____

_____

_____

_____

_____

_____

_____

A Funny Moment

It took me a while to get this one, and then I did not stop laughing for a while.

A former patient was visiting the neuro ICU as I was talking to a physical therapist who works there.

The therapist recognized the patient and called out, "Hey, stranger, so nice to see you again!"

The patient turned around and responded, "I am not stranger than I was yesterday, but it is nice to see you as well."

Neuro humor. When all else fails, laugh.

Your thoughts

The Global ICU

We live in northern Virginia, very close to Washington, DC. An inherent part of living here, and the reason we chose to live here, is the diversity of the people.

The doctors were Slovenian, Indian, American, Lebanese, among many nationalities. The nurses were Afghani, American, South African, and more.

And then one evening, at his bedside, we had friends praying and chanting and I counted seven languages. Seven different languages, but all focused on one thing: asking the Universe for healing.

A prayer in any language is a prayer. Having such a diverse group made me realize how alike we all really are and that in the end, we are all in this together.

Your thoughts

Feeding the Ones You Love

I had not realized, since I had never been in this situation before, that while I was in the ICU, my kids at home and my family and friends who were visiting and staying with us would need to be fed—in our case, for well over a month. People asked how that was going to happen, and I wasn't sure. I did not want to ask them to cook for themselves, and for us, as I felt it would be a huge obligation. I thought I would run home each morning and cook, and then come back to spend the rest of the day in the ICU. Or I might ask my older son (who was in his senior year of high school then) to cook or manage with takeout. None of those were truly viable options.

I felt worn-out, embarrassed at not being able to manage, and helpless. I was being offered assistance but could not get myself to say yes.

But our situation was dire. I could not leave the ICU, I felt, even for a moment. Anything could happen at any time.

I took the help being offered: meals, pickups, drop-offs, school trips, laundry, cleaning the house . . . I expressed gratitude. And

I prayed to be kinder to myself and those around me who needed help.

Your thoughts

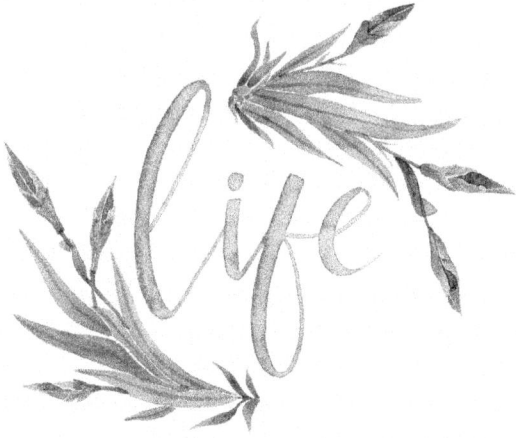

life

Darkness

I do not know how to describe the dark times in the ICU. They are different for everyone, but here is the deal: They are there for everyone. It is the ICU and things can get bad quickly.

During the darkest moments, I sit there and do the only thing I can do intentionally at that moment: I breathe. Just breathe. In and out. Slow and deep. Every part of me wants to run away, turn back the clock, shut my eyes tightly and hope that when I open them this nightmare will be over.

But the truth is, it is hard. It is here and it is, for the moment, real.

At those moments, it seems nothing brings solace except just holding the hand of the one you love, and breathing. Quietly, purposefully, peacefully.

At one point, I saw him struggling to breathe and felt this pang of guilt that I could breathe and he could not. Why?

There is no good answer to that question.

Your thoughts

Night Terrors

One night in the ICU, I could not get my system to calm down. No matter what I did, I could not seem to settle.

I was in the midst of a massive anxiety attack. I had never had one before. I did not know what was wrong. I could not catch my breath, my hands shook and I thought I would pass out.

I felt guilty even calling my own doctor to help me as I watched my husband struggling to breathe.

I had to understand, as my doctor said, that if I did not take care of myself, I would not be able to take care of my husband or my children.

I took the doctor's advice and began to take short breaks every hour—to hug my kids, to meditate, to walk, to get a cup of coffee, to breathe, and to train my brain to stop asking, *Why us?*

Your thoughts

_____

_____

_____

_____

_____

_____

_____

_____

_____

_____

_____

_____

All Humans

One day there was a lot of activity on one of the hospital floors. I saw a lot of cops. I thought for sure there was a celebrity on the floor.

Turns out it was a prisoner.

I didn't know who he was or what he had done or what was wrong with him. It just tells us how selfless humans can be to care for someone who has been incarcerated for whatever reason. They took care of him and he left in three days. (This is an assumption on my part, as the cops disappeared.)

In the hospital, you are only judged and cared for based on your illness, not who you are in the outside world. In that sense, all are treated fairly and equally.

Your thoughts

Hope

At some points in the night, I would stand next to his bed and just watch him breathe. Chest going up and down. I even placed my finger under his nose to feel the warmth of this breath. There was no other movement in his body at the time.

But, my heart believed, as long as there is breath, there is hope.

Where there is hope, there is possibility, and possibility carries happiness somewhere in its folds.

❦

Your thoughts

Energy

One evening, one of the nurses asked me if I believed in energy healing. Her question took me by surprise. Here we were in the middle of this bastion of modern medicine with what seemed to me like every high-end piece of equipment and medication known to man, and a well-trained nurse was asking me about something very New Age.

I do believe in energy healing and, honestly, if at that time she had said that if I did a hundred sun salutations every hour, he would wake up, I would have done them.

I requested that she do her healing session, and she performed several Reiki sessions for Sameer.

Now, this is not part of her job description or her duties, nor did she charge me any money. She kept saying that it was part of who she was as a healer, and healing him made her feel stronger as well. This seems to me to be the common theme in the ICU—their profession is their calling.

Your thoughts

_____

_____

_____

_____

_____

_____

_____

_____

_____

_____

_____

Bitten

One day, another nurse who had been caring for Sameer came in looking a bit off-center. This surprised me as she was one of the optimistic nurses in the ICU. Already being on pins and needles, I thought she was reacting to my husband's charts and that she knew something she wasn't telling me, so I asked her if everything was okay.

"Not really," she said with a faint smile. A patient had bit her. She had to get a shot. She still smiled and did her job and left.

It had never occurred to me that the nurses would face things like this. When we talked later, she told me she had, in her heart, forgiven the person who bit her.

Each day brings a new lesson to me. Whether I am ready to learn it or not.

Your thoughts

Bathroom Break

Around one a.m., it is quiet in the ICU. I need a bathroom break. I leave the ICU, as the bathroom is outside in the corridor.

And I am instantly locked out of the ICU. I buzz to be let in but there is no response. I sit on the cold corridor floor waiting for someone to let me in. (This happens a lot late at night and I am used to waiting.)

A young Mexican lady arrives. I know her brother is in there as well. We don't know each other's names. Just each other's pain.

She sits on the floor with me as we wait for someone to open the door. It takes a few minutes sometimes, and I reckon the people inside have more important work to do at this dreadful hour of the night.

We sit together. I share her potato chips.

The door opens. She stands up and gives me a hug and says, "You just picture him walking out of here on his own two legs. I am doing the same."

She smiles and walks away.

I am grateful for the break that came with a heaping helping of much-needed optimism.

Your thoughts

_____

_____

_____

_____

_____

_____

_____

_____

_____

_____

_____

_____

Protest

A friend reminded me to stay patient with others. I was angry at someone who was supposed to help but did not. Seems like there is always someone like that.

My friend made a sign for me and stuck it on the bottom of my water bottle: "Patience."

She reminded me again and again not to give my energy to the wrong place. Stay patient instead. Use the energy to keep myself sane. So each time someone said something that hurt—what will you do if he dies/have you looked at stem cell transplants (something he did not need)/have the doctors told you if this will recur/what quality of life will he have when he wakes up/what will your children do without a father—I would remind myself to start counting backwards from a thousand in Hindi (my mother tongue but I am terrible at numbers in Hindi, so it would really distract me). Truth be told, there were days when I would listen to these questions and the response inside my head was to come up with as many cuss words as I could recall in any language. But I chose not to react. People, it seems to me, weren't looking for answers—just reflecting my own anxiety, perhaps.

By having patience and not reacting, I was able to conserve my energy for things that mattered.

Your thoughts

_____

_____

_____

_____

_____

_____

_____

_____

_____

_____

_____

_____

Depends on the Destination

An older gentleman had, from what I could tell, been sedated for a while. After he woke up, he complained to the nurses as he had no idea where he was.

One morning I was standing outside his room as they were preparing to wheel him out on his bed. My guess is that they were taking him for some tests.

"Are you ready to go?" they asked him.

"Only if you aren't wheeling me to the morgue," he said as loudly and boldly as his frail body let him.

Your thoughts

Normal

When someone becomes critically ill, everything changes. I am not sure how things go back to the way they were before, or if they will, or if it matters if they do.

A big lesson I learned in watching my own husband and others in the ICU was that from the day they come in, there will be a new normal. One patient was admitted with severe blackouts and recovered; however, she lost one year of memory. She could remember nothing about the past year. Another patient's older spouse would ask me, every single day, if everything was going to be okay for us. Then she would say, it will never be the same no matter what. I don't know if her husband made it out. I saw one woman in the waiting room who would bring terrific healthy lunches for herself each day. I never saw her eating anything. She would place the lunch on the table. Stare at it and put it back in her bag.

A new normal.

It just is. For now. Then the cycle will change again and there will be a new, better normal.

Your thoughts

Wild Horses

I saw an old, seriously ill man being wheeled out on a gurney. And overheard him say, "When I get out of here, I am going to get myself a car that has more horsepower than the cars that are on racecourses. My car will have so much horsepower, it will be banned everywhere. That is what I am going to drive."

Life is so fucking unfair sometimes. Those who have the spirit and want to live are struggling on gurneys, and then there are so many of us with so much to be grateful for who complain about silly things like the coffee being too cold.

I never saw that old man again. I hope he got a new car.

Your thoughts

_____

_____

_____

_____

_____

_____

_____

_____

_____

_____

_____

_____

If These Walls Could Talk

Sitting inside the super-chilly ICU, I am sipping hot water from a cup to stay warm.

I look around the room. At first, I was scared to enter the ICU. It is, after all, a place where seriously ill people are housed.

But after experiencing this long stay here and being with the doctors and nurses who dedicate their lives to healing people, I have begun to think differently. I wonder how many people have sat in the same chair where I am sitting today and offered unending prayers to God/the Universe/whatever they believed in to heal their loved ones.

I begin to look at the room differently. Instead of viewing it as a place of anxiety and grief, I see at it as a place where many prayers are answered. Where the walls of the room, if they could talk, are perhaps positively influenced by the prayers of all those who sit here and wish that things will get better soon.

I see people leaving other ICU rooms surrounded by family and loads of balloons. I see the nurses smiling as serious cases turn the corner. I have started to become accustomed, as much as someone can, to my new environment.

I am sure this room has seen its share of desperation and death. But by the same token, it has seen its share of healing and miracles. I choose to believe that.

Your thoughts

A Little Knowledge

At one point, after the worst was over, my husband began to cough. It sounded nasty. I panicked. I couldn't understand why the nurses weren't getting upset that he was coughing so hard.

"His lungs are working perfectly and he will do great," they told me, but in my heart, all I could hear was a nasty cough.

I went home that night to hug the kids and have a meal with them. I remembered nights when the kids, as little babies, would have coughs. The ER visits almost always, luckily, resulted in the doctor saying that coughs sound worse than they are, and that the baby would be fine.

I smiled and went back to the hospital and tried not to cringe at the cough, but instead say to myself that his system was recovering. The other thoughts were too frightening.

Your thoughts

ICU Amnesia

There were days that I want to forget. The sounds of the machines, the smell of the medication, the look of devastation on the faces of the doctors, the round-the-clock care by the ICU staff, the explosive bowels, the neurosurgeon screaming at the top of his lungs to rouse my husband from a medical coma (this is actually a specific technique and not just yelling).

There were so many of those dark moments.

"You know, he won't remember a thing when he wakes up," one ICU nurse told me. "He won't know what happened, how bad it was, or what anyone who is here experienced."

My girlfriend who was with me at the time hugged me hard, and we both cried. Tears of joy, mostly. But deep in my heart, a bit of envy: Was there anything they could give me so my family, and I too, could forget this darkness?

I think there is something that helps: time.

It doesn't help in the moment, when everything seems to be falling apart at once. But in the long run, the Universe gives us time—which, as cliché as it sounds, does help us heal. And, eventually, forget. Or at least not remember. There is a difference.

Your thoughts

_____

_____

_____

_____

_____

_____

_____

_____

_____

_____

_____

_____

_____

Monitoring the Monitors

He has a white band on his hand. It is connected to a monitor. I believe the monitor checks his oxygen level.

The nurses say it should not go below 92.

I begin to watch it like a hawk.

96. 97. 95. 93. 92. I begin to panic. I get up to go call the nurse. Before I open the door, she is already there.

We both look at the monitor: 99. 98. 99.

They tell me not to monitor it. They are already monitoring it.

I still do. Because it is as though I am monitoring myself. It gives me something to do. If I don't look at the numbers, I have to analyze what is going on and what it means.

99. 98. 95. 93. 95.

And so it goes. On and on.

Your thoughts

_____

_____

_____

_____

_____

_____

_____

_____

_____

_____

_____

Fashion in the ICU

Sameer has been in the ICU for a month. In a coma. He now has a full beard. I tell my little one that Daddy has a beard now and he tells me it is in fashion in India, as all the cricketers have beards.

Our friends, who have been with me around the clock in the ICU, hear the little one and we all laugh together. "Daddy is more fashionable now than when he wasn't sick."

The little one hasn't seen his father for days. I worry that the sounds of the machines, the images of the tubes will give him nightmares. I hope I am making the right decision. One of Sameer's friends came by to see him and literally took a step back when he saw the tubes, the respirator and all the machines that were keeping Sameer alive. I couldn't get myself to bring my really young child into this room. He comes to visit every day, but only as far as the waiting room. Soon, I know, he will be able to see his father and his father will be well. With a very fashionable beard.

Your thoughts

_____

_____

_____

_____

_____

_____

_____

_____

_____

_____

_____

_____

The Body Does What the Body Does!

There was an older cantankerous gentleman in one of the rooms in the ICU. Whenever I passed his room, I would hear him complaining to the nurses. Most of the complaints were heartbreaking. For the life of him, he could not understand why he was in the ICU or why he had all the tubes going in and out of him. I am not a doctor or a medical professional, so I won't even attempt to guess at his illness, but suffice it to say that he seemed to be lost.

One afternoon, as I was passing, I heard him say, "One day. Just for one day can you forget about doing this to me? JUST ONE DAY?"

The nurse's answer: "Mr. D., I am sorry, but everyone has bowel movements."

It was the first time I heard the old man laughing. The nurse and the tech in the room laughed. For one moment, it was okay. They were all in it together.

Your thoughts

Bite-Sized Blessings

A close friend of ours came by on many days with lunch for us. She would bring in food, place napkins on the cafeteria table, set out plastic knives and forks. Try to make it look as appetizing as possible.

A few days I could eat. Most days, I stared at the food. He was in a coma. How do you nurture yourself when the one you love cannot eat?

Then my kids would join us and would not eat until I ate.

The Universe has its ways. I don't always understand them, but learned to let go and be guided by what I needed to do more than what I was expected to do or what I thought I should do.

I needed to eat to survive to take care of my family.

At first, each bite brought guilt. Then I learned to be grateful. I had a friend feeding me and my spirit.

Your thoughts

It Is Always the Food

There was a sign at the hospital for a very important meeting. It was a meeting for the hospital staff to discuss some essential issues. I remember seeing that sign almost every day for about two weeks.

All I remember from the sign is that at the bottom was a line that read: "There will be food and wine. Free."

I had to laugh. My family's entire experience at the hospital was about life and death, about machines and medicines, about doctors and nurses. I had forgotten that normal situations existed—even in an intense hospital.

Your thoughts

Why Me?

It never occurs to me—which in itself is weird—that the first thing he will want to know when he wakes up is why it happened to him.

Why me?

As I sit here in the ICU and look at his struggling chest, the tubes that help him breathe, I would give anything to hear him utter any words.

I just did not think the words would be, *Why me?*

Because, I guess, it is another thing that I have no answer to. I don't know that anyone really does.

I was talking to one of his therapists, who said the only way to answer that question is to ask, *Why not me?*

It is a tough one. I don't know that there is a right answer, or more aptly a satisfying answer, to either of those questions.

I am grateful that he is here to ask it.

Your thoughts

_____

_____

_____

_____

_____

_____

_____

_____

_____

_____

_____

_____

What Matters

I overhear the nurses in the cafeteria one day discussing the cost of living in this area.

"I used to work at a funeral home and made no money. So I became a nurse," one says.

"Nursing pays more?" asks the other one.

"No, but at least I can pay my loans now knowing that I am helping people live instead of focusing on dead people."

Your thoughts

The "No Crying" Rule

I had my own rule for the ICU room. I am not sure it will make sense to anyone, so hear me out.

Perhaps, being influenced by Hollywood and Bollywood, I have this theory that people in a coma can hear.

I don't truly know if he can hear us or not, but my rule, based on that theory, was simple: no crying in the ICU and no talking about how bad things are.

Everyone who came in had to sit down and tell us good stories, good memories they shared with him.

A dear friend pulled out her iPhone and read stories about Spain to my husband, as Spain is one of his favorite places.

I don't know if he heard or if it made a difference to him, but I can tell you it made a difference to us. Each story reminded us who we were fighting for: a loved one who is a great father, a fantastic friend, a funny storyteller, and a kind husband. *He is not just a patient.* He is a person with a story, with many stories.

Outside the ICU, we wept as we held each other. Then once inside, we only talked about and envisioned a healthy future. For his sake—and I have to admit, for ours.

Your thoughts

In the Darkness

Everything I stood for came to a head one night when things just kept going from bad to worse. One of the medical staff members asked me if I understood that he may never wake up and that they had done all they could.

"This may be as well as he gets," she said, pointing to my husband's totally paralyzed body lying helplessly on the hospital bed.

It was then I realized what faith truly means.

I had thought the worst might happen, and I understood—in my brain. But my heart never accepted that fact. If miracles happen every day, why wouldn't they happen with us?

I chose to believe we would walk out of there together.

It was a thought by choice. I was trying not to let the demons in my own mind win.

Your thoughts

The Moment

After he woke from the coma, it was decided they would use a speech valve to see if he could speak and if his vocal chords were okay.

The therapist placed the valve, then asked my husband for his name. We waited, holding our breaths. He answered correctly.

The next question: "Where do you live?"

Answer: "Hospital."

The therapist looked at me and said, "Well, technically, he isn't wrong."

The moment is the lifetime? Right?

Your thoughts

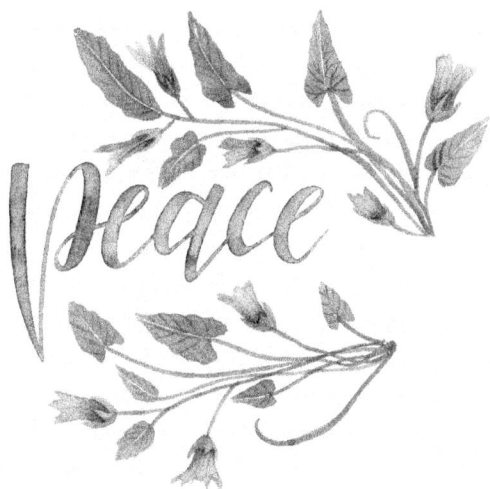

peace

Movement

He isn't moving due to the medical coma.

Then suddenly, he starts shivering, badly. I worry but am happy that he is showing movement.

The doctors, really worried, give him medication to stop the shivering. To stop the movement.

He lies completely paralyzed again. Then the worry that he is not moving returns.

The paradox of healing.

Learning to trust the medicine men.

Your thoughts

_____

_____

_____

_____

_____

_____

_____

_____

_____

_____

_____

Why Walk?

"Sir, we will have you walking in no time," the physical therapist says to the old man in the wheelchair as he eats his mac and cheese.

"But I don't want to walk," he replies.

"Why?"

"Because I want to dance."

I run back into the room to tell my husband. I reach the room and stop at the door. The doctors are busy discussing his latest CT scan and a new lifesaving procedure.

"You will dance, someday," I whisper as I stand on the sidelines.

No one hears me.

Your thoughts

The World We Live In

I don't know his passwords. Bills are due. He pays the bills. How do I leave and go to the bank to pay bills?

The text messages are about the toilet overflowing, a friend needs help with a problem, a relative loses a job.

The doctors say the medications don't seem to be working.

I look at my phone. The outside world needs attention.

All together now. How do we do it all?

I turn my phone off.

It can all wait for today.

Your thoughts

_____

_____

_____

_____

_____

_____

_____

_____

_____

_____

_____

_____

When Rules Don't Matter

After he woke from the illness, I was sitting by his bedside. He looked around and said to me, "I am lost."

All I could think of was, *So am I.*

I told him what had happened and where he had been, what was going on, and how well he was healing.

He nodded, closed his eyes, and went back to sleep.

I stood there. Clutching myself.

I broke my own rule and wept in the ICU.

Your thoughts

_____

_____

_____

_____

_____

_____

_____

_____

_____

_____

_____

_____

_____

The Meaning Is Yours

There is a tech who has a tattoo of teardrops on the side of her face. I ask her what they mean. "The teardrops remind me of the ones I love and they allow my sorrow to flow."

Beauty is everywhere.

Your thoughts

One Sock at a Time

A woman is learning to walk. The therapist keeps dropping socks in front of her so she can learn to walk and bend down and pick up something.

After picking up about ten socks, the exasperated patient says to the therapist: "Can you at least throw something worth picking up?"

I watch in envy. I would be happy for him to walk and pick up anything.

He is awake. He recognizes us. He knows who he is. No memory loss, he can hug his kids, he can laugh. We've gotten this far. It will be a matter of time before he is picking up socks.

Your thoughts

Who Is Ill?

"I want to tell you something important. My husband got a tumor when he was young. It was benign and it was removed. But it affected him because it was near his ear and he was a musician." An older woman I met at the time is telling me her story about her husband's journey through a difficult illness. She talks about how hard his recovery was and how it affected his ability as a musician. The tumor that didn't kill him to some extent destroyed his identity. He had to find his place in the world again. She was not the wife of a musician anymore. They had to get used to a new normal.

"Here is what I want you to know: When your spouse gets ill, it affects everyone. It has been twenty years since his tumor surgery, and to this day we refer to it as 'our tumor.'"

I hug her, and she soothes my tears as I weep for us.

Your thoughts

How Do You Do It?

Sometimes patients (and their families) are upset, and I see them getting angry at the staff, I see patients crying, I see them struggling. The nurses see it all and try to work through it. How, how do they do this day in and day out?

"I don't serve people. I serve God. And not the God in temples and churches. I serve the God of love. To me God is love. So I do this for love. If I do it for any other reason, I won't survive," the nurse tells me. I have seen the pain in her eyes as she helps the patients. It is real. It has to be love. How else can they do this?

Your thoughts

Ice Packs

You never know what tips you will learn from the nursing staff. One day, the nurse hears me talking to my older son who has hurt himself on the soccer field. I am telling him to ice his knee using the packet of frozen peas in the freezer.

"I'll let you in on a secret. I have many kids and they are always using frozen food like that. I never know which one has been used and put back. And I don't want them to use it and put it back and then I cook it. So here is my secret: I buy bags of lima beans. I know *no one* in my family eats those, so those are their ice packs. Keeps my peas safe for cooking."

The next day, I have my son buy bags of frozen lima beans, as I am reminded that I am not just a caregiver for my husband, but also for my young sons.

Your thoughts

_____

_____

_____

_____

_____

_____

_____

_____

_____

_____

_____

_____

How to Heal

A friend of mine, who can only be described as a genius, says to my husband: "There is one prerequisite to healing. It is not the doctors, the nurses, the machines, the medication. All that will come after. The most important thing: Start to believe you can get better. Then it will all help."

I want to ask, *What happens if you believe and it doesn't work?* I stop myself. If I ask that, then I am implying that my belief isn't 100 percent true. That I have some doubt somewhere.

I try consciously to practice belief, but it seems forced. I try saying it out loud as an affirmation, and the words sound hollow to my own ears. *I BELIEVE.*

Then, I try writing it out: *I believe he will heal. I believe all will be well.*

The writing seems to help me. Writing down every day what I am grateful for now and what I will be grateful for in the future. My belief that all will be well.

Even as I write in my journal, I console myself that being a believer 100 percent of the time is hard to put into practice, but not doing so is not an option I want to explore.

Your thoughts

Hiding in Plain Sight

I am walking to my husband's room and I see a patient on a walker and his nurse in the hallway. Suddenly he pulls the nurse back and they move behind a wall.

I am pretty close to them and hear him say, "Just stay put here for a second. My ex works here and I can see her standing at the counter."

I laugh, but I am not sure the nurse is amused.

❦

Your thoughts

Finding Peace

Why did this happen to him?

Why did this happen to us?

Why does this happen to anyone?

I am told, and I think a part of me understands, that there really is no good answer to those questions.

Then a friend of mine, who is an attorney, says to me: "You can keep asking these questions, trying to see if you find answers that satisfy you. But here is my truth: You will find true peace when you transcend the questions."

He is right. I am not ready yet. I hope some day I will be.

Some day soon.

Very soon.

Your thoughts

This and Only This

A text from a friend who is a caregiver for a chronically ill child: "One day today will be in the past. You will get through this. It will pass. The pain seems unbearable, I know. But I have learned that the painful moments do pass, even though they seem like they will stay forever."

It is the only law of nature I believe in 1,000 percent. Everything passes. Good, bad, or otherwise.

It will pass.

It will.

Your thoughts

The Three Ladies of Fate

A friend who loves mythology visits the ICU and tell me about the three ladies of fate in Greek mythology: One spins the thread of life, the second measures that thread, and then the third one snips it. In this way, they determine how long someone will live and when they are going to die.

He sees the grief on my face and says: "I am not telling you this to scare you. I am telling you this to make you understand that even in the olden days, people understood that certain things are out of our control. We can only control our reactions, and nothing else."

I cannot tell you how many versions of this I heard in the months at the hospital, and even during his many months of postoperative care.

It isn't the easiest thing to swallow. As a recovering engineer, my instinct is to try to fix everything. As a working writer, I think it is my job to observe it, become aware of it, and learn from it. As a human being, I want to scream. If nothing is under our control, then what is the point of everything? Why plan? Why not just give in to destiny?

I struggle with accepting the idea of fate and destiny versus creating our own path in life.

Your thoughts

True Sight

When nothing seemed to be working right, I reminded myself of the words of Derek Rydall: "Let yourself be led by insight and not by eyesight." (I remember hearing him on a podcast; he has some terrific books out as well, if you are interested.)

I'd leave the ICU, go for a walk. I'd offer prayers. I'd try to meditate. I knew that my instincts were strong, but overpowered by the harsh reality coming at all my senses. I couldn't make sense of all the darkness in front of my eyes, so I focused on the simple art of just getting up and leaving for a few minutes, walking and just being, without worrying about every single thing. It helped me to come back refreshed to try again.

Lather, rinse, repeat.

Your thoughts

_____

_____

_____

_____

_____

_____

_____

_____

_____

_____

_____

_____

The Hands

One of the nurses explained to me the difference between her and a caregiver (usually a spouse, a friend, a companion, a relative).

"We have been blessed with caring hands. You have been blessed with loving hands. A patient needs both to survive and thrive."

She explains the difference in recovery rates of patients who have family visit them versus the ones who have no one. I have seen it myself—there is one patient who refuses to eat because she is all alone and no one ever visits. I see the nurses go in and sit and eat with her, but she refuses to touch her food. I overhear the nurses worry about what will happen when she is released. There may be no one to take her home.

"What do I have to live for?" the patient says so many times. Her room is right across the corridor. I hear her painful cries.

Your thoughts

Of Curses and Blessings

I was buying a chocolate bar (yes, it helps) from the hospital gift shop when I heard the old white-haired Indian man who volunteers as the cashier tell this story. He was telling the story to his coworker, but when he saw me listening, he included me.

I am paraphrasing here and any error is mine.

"A man is told by a doctor that he has a massive tumor and he has only six months to live. The man decides that if he has only six months to live, he will do what he can to make his life happy and to complete what he considered his calling. He wanted to paint his church. The church was up on a hill and the man was frail and poor. So he decided that every day, he would carry one pail of paint up the hill to the church and paint. Every day, he walked up the church. He said his prayers, he was grateful for one more day to paint. He drank water, ate simple meals, and painted. As he saw the walls filling with color, his heart rejoiced.

"Each day he made the difficult trek. Up the hill. Down the hill. His heart filled with joy that he was filling his life's purpose.

"He carried the paint up and down the hill. First one pail, then more. He felt himself getting stronger.

"Six months later, he was still alive. The church was still in need of paint.

"The man lived, tumor-free, and the church radiated beautiful colors."

The point, the old man told me, was that it was important not to let the obstacles get in the way of your true calling, and to be grateful every day. "Who knows how he was cured—maybe it was the exercise of going up and down the hill, maybe it was what he ate when he was there, maybe it was just the will to live. The point is, he was grateful and happy for what he had and did not focus on what he did not have."

Your thoughts

What Do You See?

As we waited for the surgeon to tell us what was going on this time around, my friend Brian sat by my side. We were discussing the power of intention. I am a stronger believer in intent and was trying hard to hold a positive intent but, honestly, the devastating situation at hand seemed to be winning over my mind.

Brian, who is also a strong believer in intent, shared this interesting story with me. He reminded me of a tragic shooting spree that happened in our area a few years ago. The only clue the police had was that the shooters were in a white van.

What happened next in that case, Brian told me, shows us that we see what we are looking for—people everywhere began to notice white vans, and boy, there were a LOT of white vans on the street.

He asked me to look around and see how many people were holding a certain type of coffee mug. And in the nine hours we sat in the waiting room, I saw so many people with the exact same mug.

Brian reminded me to set my intentions to see the small blessings instead of the enormous obstacles in my way.

This isn't just some "be happy" hokeypokey. Trust me, some days were so hard, I was tempted to say *Fuck it all, I give up. This is so bad. I cannot do anything.* And those were the days I needed to set my intentions the most. If the only thing I was grateful for was that the water fountain was working, so be it. Every breath was hope, every movement meant there was yet a chance he could walk out. It meant another day to hope and another moment to see things change for the better.

Your thoughts

_____

_____

_____

_____

_____

_____

_____

_____

_____

_____

_____

Best Blessing Ever

I was raised in a culture where adults often place their hands on their children's heads (or on the heads of younger people) and offer blessings: live long and prosper, may you be blessed with great health, and so on.

Those blessings have always provided great comfort.

During the time at the ICU, our family became close to a friend who is a famous attorney. He is Indian by birth. Every time he texted me to offer support, or showed up to help, or emailed me, his message always ended with the same blessing: *Khush Raho* (always be happy).

At first, I found the blessing strange. Shouldn't the blessing be about health and well-being?

Then, after things calmed down, I realized what he was trying to say: That at the end of it all, all we really want is happiness (some call it peace). I realized his blessing meant that I should try to be happy now. That was all that mattered. Tomorrow may or may not come, and who knows what it will bring. In addition, I feel like other blessings lead to the same end point: happiness.

So at the end of this book, I leave you with the same blessing: No matter what you are facing, no matter where you are and what life hands you, *Khush Raho*. May you always be happy and have peace.

Your thoughts

_____

_____

_____

_____

_____

_____

_____

_____

_____

_____

_____

_____

_____

Check Out

The day Sameer was to be released from the hospital, my sister and I went to the cafeteria to grab a quick bite.

The lady at the checkout counter had been talking to us for weeks now. That day, my sister said to her, "We are leaving now. This will be our last meal here."

The lady smiled, gave us our check, and said, "I hope whatever was broken is fixed now."

The best blessings come at the most unexpected moments.

Your thoughts

_____

_____

_____

_____

_____

_____

_____

_____

_____

_____

_____

_____

Resources

1. The American Stroke Association has a lot of helpful information on their site.

2. Many hospitals have free support groups. Do check them out if you can.

3. Most big hospitals have quiet areas for prayer. Just sitting in those areas, free of all the noise of the hospital, is quite helpful.

4. There are so many books on caregiving. I am hard-pressed to name just one. They do help. If nothing else, they make us understand that we are not alone.

5. Our local government has a lot of resources for people who find themselves in a medical crisis. Be sure to check your local government website for help.

6. In the US, illness brings with it a ton of paperwork. Recruit a friend/family member/trusted person to help with it (should you need the help). It can get overwhelming quickly.

Acknowledgements

To all our friends, family, doctors, nurses, techs, and even complete strangers who helped us during this devastating time: thank you so much. There is something magical when a community comes together to save someone. And we are blessed to have been the recipients of such magic.

Thank you, all.

To my team who helped this book come alive: thank you! Jennifer Lawler, Suzanne Fass, Simi Jois, Paayal Sharma, Ramin Ganeshram, Betty-Ann Quirino, Popsy Kangaratnam, Luca Marchiori, Ana Di, Linda Whittig, Amy Riolo, Niv Mani, Aviva Goldfarb, Mollie Cox Bryan, Sangeeta Bongmom, Jenni Field and Stephanie Caruso—this could not have been possible without your support. I am so grateful to you all.

About the Author

Monica Bhide is an award-winning writer, accomplished literary coach, gifted poet, storyteller, and educator with a lyrical voice and universal appeal. As a bestselling fiction and internationally renowned cookbook author, Monica is known for sharing food, culture, mystery, and love in her writing. Having roots and experience in many places, Monica inspires readers everywhere with present-day stories that transcend cultural, chronological, geographical, economical, and religious borders.

A respected writing authority, Monica appears regularly on NPR and conducts sold-out workshops on writing, food, culture, and scheduled speaking events at such prestigious venues as the Smithsonian Institution, Sackler Gallery, Les Dames d'Escoffier, Georgetown University, and Yale University. She has taught all over the world, including conferences in London, Dubai, the US, and more.

As a noted international food writer, Monica has built a diverse and solid audience through her books and articles in top-tier media such as: *The New York Times, The Washington Post, Ladies Home Journal, AARP—the Magazine, Parents, Chicago Tribune,*

Christian Science Monitor, *Bon Appétit*, *Town and Country Travel*, *Food and Wine*, *Cooking Light*, *Coastal Living*, *Health*, *Better Nutrition*, and many others.

Monica is a graduate of George Washington University (Washington, DC), and holds a master's degree from Lynchburg College (Lynchburg, VA) and a bachelor's degree from Bangalore University (Bangalore, India). She feels fortunate for her rich, multicultural education and enjoys giving back to the global community by serving on committees and volunteering for Les Dames d'Escoffier, the International Association of Culinary Professionals, and at her children's schools in Northern Virginia.

Monica lives in Virginia with her husband and two sons.

Also by Monica Bhide

Fiction and Short Stories

Mother, a short story (Bodes Well Publishing, 2017)

Karma and the Art of Butter Chicken (Bodes Well Publishing, 2016)

The Devil In Us (2014)

Singapore Noir, edited by Cheryl Lu-Lien Tan (Akashic Books, 2014)

Food Essays and Cookbooks

A Life of Spice (2015)

Modern Spice: Inspired Indian Flavors for the Contemporary Kitchen (Simon and Schuster. 2009; Random House India, 2010)

The Everything Indian Cookbook: 300 Tantalizing Recipes from Sizzling Tandoor Chicken to Fiery Lamb Vindaloo (Adams Media, 2004)

Monica's essays have been included in *Best Food Writing 2005*, *2009*, *2010,* and *2014*, edited by Holly Hughes (Da Capo Press)

Inspirational Books

In Conversation with Exceptional Women (ebook)

Poetry

Telltales (Bodes Well Publishing, 2017, ebook)

Monica's books are available through Amazon.com, BN.com, Kobo, iBooks and her website, MonicaBhide.com.

www.ingramcontent.com/pod-product-compliance
Lightning Source LLC
Chambersburg PA
CBHW051954090426
42741CB00008B/1391